STAY HEALTHY

AN ALL WEATHER GUIDE

CYRIL LAKES

Contents

CHAPTER ONE

INTRODUCTION

"Stay healthy" is a motto for living a fulfilling life, not merely a catchphrase. Being well is crucial for reaching our objectives, following our passions, and living life to the fullest in the fast-paced world of today. How can we, however, "stay healthy," and what does this mean?

Maintaining one's health requires a comprehensive approach to wellbeing that takes into account one's mental, emotional, and physical well-being. It's about providing our bodies with wholesome food, working out frequently, making rest and sleep a priority, efficiently handling stress, and cultivating wholesome connections and relationships.

This introduction to maintaining your health will cover the essential elements of wellbeing and offer helpful advice and methods for implementing healthy routines into your everyday life. This book will give you the information and resources you need to stay healthy and prosper, whether your goals are to strengthen your immune system, maintain a healthy weight, increase your level of exercise, or improve your general quality of life.

Come along with us as we explore the transformational power of living a balanced and full life, the significance of self-care, and the power of good habits in the pursuit of optimal health and well-being. By working together, we may give ourselves the power to make wise decisions and design a lively, robust, and vital life.

What is meant by "wellness" and "health"

Physical, mental, emotional, and social components of well-being are all included in the concept of health and wellbeing. Despite their frequent interchange, the terms "health" and "wellness" have different meanings:

The term "health" describes the whole state of a person's physical, mental, and social well-being; it includes both the presence of positive qualities that support vitality and quality of life as well as the absence of illness or disease. It includes a range of dimensions, such as:

Physical Health: The state of the body and its physiological processes are related to physical health. It includes things like degree of fitness, diet, quality of sleep, and lack of illness or injury.

Mental Health: Mental health is the state of being emotionally and psychologically well, encompassing traits like resilience, stress management, coping mechanisms, and the capacity to uphold healthy relationships.

Social Health: The state of a person's relationships, social support systems, and sense of community belonging are all considered aspects of their social health. It involves elements like interpersonal relationships, communication abilities, and community involvement.

Wellness: Proactive efforts to maximize health and improve general well-being are the focus of wellness, which extends beyond the absence of illness. It entails actively partaking in actions and routines that support mental, emotional, and physical health as well as a sense of contentment and life's meaning. There are several facets to wellness, such as:

Physical wellbeing: Maintaining physical wellbeing is taking good care of one's body by consistent exercise, a healthy diet, enough sleep, and preventative medical procedures. It places a strong emphasis on preserving ideal levels of energy and physical fitness.

Emotional Wellbeing: This refers to the ability to recognize and control one's feelings, build resilience, and maintain an optimistic attitude on life. It entails techniques like mindfulness, stress management, self-care, and asking for help when necessary.

Building and maintaining wholesome connections, encouraging a feeling of connection and belonging, and improving the wellbeing of others within communities are all important aspects of social wellness. Effective communication, empathy, teamwork, and social interaction are all necessary.

All things considered, wellness and health are related ideas that cover comprehensive well-being in all domains physical, mental, emotional, and social. Individuals can live happy, fulfilled lives and reach their full potential in all facets of life by placing a high priority on their health and fitness.

Proper Nutrition and Eating Practices

Promoting general health and well-being is largely dependent on nutrition and good eating practices. Our bodies can be supported in maintaining physical vitality, cognitive function, emotional stability, and illness prevention by feeding them a well-balanced diet full of important nutrients. The following are some fundamentals of nutrition and sensible eating practices:

Dietary Balance: Try to eat a varied range of nutrient-dense foods from every food group in a balanced diet. Fruits, vegetables, whole grains, lean meats, and good fats are all included in this. For optimum health, each food group offers crucial vitamins, minerals, antioxidants, and other nutrients.

Portion Control: To prevent overindulging, be careful of portion sizes and consume in moderation. Avoid consuming excessive portions and pay attention to the serving sizes that are suggested for various food groups, particularly when dining out or consuming packaged meals.

A colorful plate should have a range of vibrant fruits and vegetables on it. These foods are high in antioxidants, fiber, vitamins, and minerals. In order to make sure you're getting a variety of nutrients, try to incorporate a rainbow of colors into your meals.

Whole Foods: Whenever feasible, opt for whole, minimally processed foods. Nutrient-dense whole foods fruits, vegetables, whole grains, legumes, nuts, seeds, and lean proteins acquire vital nutrients in their unaltered states without the need for additional sweets, bad fats, or preservatives.

Eat Less Processed Foods and Added Sugars: Reduce the amount of foods and drinks that are heavy in harmful fats, processed carbs, and added sugars. These consist of processed snacks, sugar-filled beverages, desserts, candies, fried foods, and high-calorie, low-nutrient foods. Choose complete, nutrient-dense substitutes instead.

Good Fats: Include foods like avocados, nuts, seeds, olive oil, fatty fish (including salmon, mackerel, and sardines), flaxseeds, and nuts and seeds in your diet. Hormone production, cognitive function, and the absorption of fat-soluble vitamins all depend on healthy fats.

Hydration: Throughout the day, make sure you drink lots of water to stay hydrated. Water is necessary for several body processes, including as digestion, the absorption of nutrients, the regulation of body temperature, and the removal of toxins. Reduce your intake of sweetened beverages and replace them with infused water, herbal teas, or water.

Eating with awareness: Engage in mindful eating by being aware of your body's signals of hunger and fullness, enjoying the tastes and textures of your meal, and chewing slowly and deliberately. When eating, stay away from distractions like television or electronics and pay attention to your body's signals of hunger and fullness.

Meal Planning and Preparation: Make sure you have wholesome options on hand by planning and preparing meals in advance. Throughout the week, maintaining good eating habits and avoiding impulsive food choices can be facilitated by batch cooking, meal planning, and keeping wholesome snacks readily available.

Seek Professional Advice: For individualized advice and recommendations catered to your unique requirements, think about speaking with a licensed dietitian or nutritionist if you have any specific dietary demands, medical issues, or nutritional goals.

You may fuel your body, support optimal health and well-being, and get the advantages of a balanced and nutritious diet by embracing these nutritional guidelines and good eating practices. Keep in mind that over time, minor, sustainable adjustments can have a big impact on your general health and quality of life.

Exercise and physical activity are crucial parts of a healthy lifestyle because they improve general health and lower the risk of chronic illnesses. Include regular exercise in your regimen for a host of psychological, emotional, and physical advantages. Here are some reasons why it's crucial to engage in physical activity and some tips for doing so:

Advantages for Physical Health:

Weight management: By boosting metabolism and burning calories, regular exercise helps regulate body weight.

Cardiovascular Health: Exercise lowers the risk of high blood pressure, heart disease, and stroke by strengthening the heart and enhancing circulation.

Strength and Endurance: Strength training activities improve physical performance and lower the risk of injury by increasing muscular mass, strength, and endurance.

Bone Health: Weight-bearing activities that lower the risk of osteoporosis and maintain bone density include jogging, strength training, and walking.

Regular moderate-intensity exercise has been demonstrated to strengthen the immune system and lower the risk of infection.

Advantages for the Mind and Emotion:

Stress Reduction: Engaging in physical activity triggers the brain's natural stress-relieving chemicals, endorphins, to be released. This promotes relaxation and lowers anxiety and depressive symptoms.

Enhanced Mood: Engaging in physical activity raises levels of neurotransmitters like dopamine and serotonin, which in turn promote emotions of happiness and wellbeing.

Improved Sleep Quality: Frequent exercise helps people fall asleep more quickly and experience deeper, more restorative sleep. It also improves the length and quality of sleep.

Improved Mental Capacity:

Brain Health: By fostering neuroplasticity the brain's capacity to adapt and reorganize in response to stimuli exercise enhances cognitive performance and guards against age-related cognitive decline.

Memory and Learning: Research has indicated a connection between physical activity and enhanced cognitive function, memory, and learning in both children and adults.

Social Advantages:

Community Engagement: Taking part in team sports, fitness courses, or leisure activities with others creates a sense of community and strengthens social relationships.

CHAPTER TWO

Exercise with friends, family, or workout partners offers accountability and support, which makes it simpler to maintain a regular exercise schedule.

Including exercise in your everyday routine doesn't have to be difficult. Aim for 75 minutes of vigorous-intensity aerobic activity or at least 150 minutes of moderate-intensity aerobic activity per week, in addition to two or more days of muscle-strengthening activities. Here are some pointers to get you going and keep you moving:

Whether it's cycling, swimming, dAancing, walking, jogging, or sports, pick things you enjoy doing.

Take brief breaks throughout the day to engage in activities to break up extended periods of sitting.

To keep yourself motivated, set attainable objectives and monitor your progress.

Include physical activity in your daily routine and make it a priority.

Look for opportunities to move during the day, such walking or biking instead of driving, or using the stairs instead of the elevator.

Pay attention to your body and select safe and suitable exercises based on your current level of fitness.

Before beginning a new fitness regimen, speak with a healthcare provider, particularly if you have any underlying medical illnesses or concerns.

You may raise your quality of life overall, improve your health, and elevate your mood by engaging in regular physical activity. Always keep in mind that even a small amount of movement matters, so pick things you enjoy doing and give them top importance for your health.

Stress Reduction and Mental Health

Keeping one's general health and mental well-being intact requires effective stress management. Stress is a typical occurrence in the fast-paced world of today, and if it is not properly controlled, it can have serious negative effects on mental health. Through the implementation of stress management techniques and prioritizing mental health, individuals can augment their resilience, mitigate the likelihood of mental health issues, and elevate their standard of living. The following are some essential ideas for reducing stress and fostering mental health:

Awareness and Recognition: Acknowledging the existence of stress and pinpointing its causes is the first step towards managing it. Keep an eye out for behavioral, emotional, and physical indicators of stress, such as tenseness in the muscles, agitation, changes in appetite, and trouble focusing. Recognizing your stressors will enable you to create useful coping mechanisms.

Develop constructive coping strategies to handle stress and increase resilience. This could involve methods of relaxation including progressive muscular relaxation, deep breathing, mindfulness exercises, or meditation. Enjoyable pursuits like hobbies, physical activity, being outside, or spending time with loved ones can all aid in lowering stress and elevating mood.

Physical Activity: Engaging in regular physical activity can help manage stress and improve mental health. Exercise promotes the release of endorphins, which are brain chemicals that naturally elevate mood and help lower levels of stress hormones like cortisol. Every day of the week, try to get in at least 30 minutes of moderate-intense exercise to boost your physical and emotional well-being.

Adopt healthy lifestyle practices that promote mental health, such as eating a balanced diet, getting enough sleep, and using less alcohol and caffeine. In addition to providing vital nutrients for brain health, a balanced diet full of fruits, vegetables, whole grains, lean meats, and healthy fats also helps control mood and energy levels.

Social Support: When under stress, make sure you have a strong social network and ask friends, family, or support groups for assistance. Speaking with reliable people about your emotions and experiences can offer perspective, emotional affirmation, and useful assistance. Spending time with loved ones and interacting with others fosters a sense of connection and belonging, both of which are critical for mental health.

Time management and task prioritization: To lessen emotions of stress and overwhelm, efficiently manage your time. Assign duties as needed, establish reasonable goals, and divide work into smaller, more manageable chunks. Maintaining a good work-life balance and avoiding burnout can also be achieved by learning to say no to extra commitments and set boundaries.

Positivity and Mindset: Develop a positive outlook and engage in self-acceptance, self-compassion, and self-compassion exercises. By rephrasing unfavorable ideas in a more realistic and balanced manner, you can counter cognitive distortions and negative thoughts. To stay present and grounded in the present, practice mindfulness and put an emphasis on positivity, gratitude, and resilience.

Seeking Professional Assistance: Do not be reluctant to seek professional assistance from a therapist, counselor, or mental health professional if stress becomes too much to handle or interferes with day-to-day functioning.

Counseling can offer helpful support, direction, and coping mechanisms to help with stress management and mental health enhancement.

By implementing these techniques into your everyday routine, you can improve mental health, manage stress, and develop resilience to face obstacles in life more confidently and easily. Recall that putting mental health and self-care first is crucial for general wellbeing and a high quality of life.

Rest and Sleep in Quality

A good night's sleep is vital for maintaining general health and wellbeing since it is important for proper mental, emotional, and physical development. Numerous biological activities, such as immune system performance, hormone balance, cognitive function, mood modulation, and general cellular repair and rejuvenation, are supported by getting enough restful sleep. The following are some essential guidelines for getting restful sleep:

Regular Sleep routine: Even on weekends, keep a regular sleep routine by going to bed and waking up at the same times each day. This enhances the quality and length of your sleep by regulating the circadian rhythm, your body's internal clock.

Establish a Calm and Comfortable Sleep Environment: Establish a calm and supportive sleep environment that encourages restfulness and relaxation. Make sure your bedroom is cold, quiet, and dark, and make sure your mattress, pillows, and bedding are comfy. To drown out distracting sounds or lights, try earplugs, blackout curtains, or white noise machines.

Create a Nightly habit: To let your body know when it's time to wind down and get ready for sleep, create a calming nightly habit. This could involve doing things like reading a book, listening to relaxing music, taking a warm bath, or practicing relaxation techniques like meditation or deep breathing.

Reduce Screen Time: Before going to bed, try to avoid spending too much time in front of computers, cellphones, tablets, and TVs. This is because the blue light these gadgets emit can disrupt the body's natural production of melatonin, a hormone that controls sleep-wake cycles. Try to switch off electronics at least an hour before going to bed and substitute screen-free activities.

Mindful Eating and Drinking: Pay attention to how you eat and how much you drink, especially in the hours before bed. Before going to bed, stay away from large meals, coffee, nicotine, and alcohol as these might cause sleep disturbances and restless or interrupted sleep.

Frequent Exercise: Getting regular exercise during the day can assist to improve the length and quality of your sleep. Most days of the week, try to get in at least 30 minutes of moderate-intensity activity. However, stay away from intense exercise right before bed as it can keep you up and make it difficult to fall asleep.

Handle Stress: To lower stress levels and encourage relaxation before bed, try stress-reduction methods including deep breathing, journaling, mindfulness meditation, or relaxation exercises. Sleep disruption caused by stress can be avoided by developing appropriate coping strategies.

Limit Naps: Excessive or prolonged napping might interfere with sleep patterns at night, even if brief naps can be helpful for some people, particularly if they're feeling tired during the day. If you must snooze, try to schedule quick power naps (20–30 minutes) early in the day to prevent disrupting your sleep at night.

Seek Professional Assistance if Needed: You should think about getting professional assistance from a healthcare provider or sleep specialist if you still have trouble falling asleep even after adopting healthy sleep habits, or if you exhibit symptoms of a sleep disorder like insomnia, sleep apnea, or restless legs syndrome. They are able to assess your sleeping habits, pinpoint underlying problems, and suggest suitable courses of action.

You may encourage healthier sleep patterns, improve general wellbeing, and take advantage of the numerous advantages of restorative sleep by making quality sleep a priority and implementing these techniques into your daily routine. Recall that getting enough sleep is crucial for maintaining a healthy lifestyle and that getting enough good sleep is necessary for optimum health and energy.

Drinking enough water and being healthy

A important component of wellness, hydration is essential for preserving general health and energy. Water is essential to our bodies for many physiological processes, such as digestion, detoxification, temperature regulation, nutrient delivery, and cellular metabolism. For the best possible state of physical, mental, and emotional health, one must drink enough water. The following are some fundamental ideas about water and its significance for health:

Hydration and Physical Well-Being:

Fluid Balance: Staying properly hydrated promotes the body's fluid balance, which in turn keeps cells, tissues, and organs operating at their best. Water cools the body, lubricates joints, and provides tissue and organ cushioning.

Water promotes healthy nutrient absorption and metabolism by making it easier for nutrients, electrolytes, and oxygen to reach cells and tissues.

Detoxification: Drinking enough water helps the kidneys work properly and aids in the removal of waste and toxins from the body through the urine.

Metabolism and Digestion: Water facilitates the breakdown of food and the absorption of nutrients during healthy digestion. Additionally, hydration promotes cell energy synthesis and metabolic functions.

Drinking enough water and being mentally well:

Cognitive Function: Sustaining alertness, focus, and cognitive function depends on enough water. Dehydration can affect mood, memory, and cognitive function, resulting in weariness, irritation, and trouble concentrating.

Mood Regulation: Emotional health and mood regulation are influenced by hydration. Research has indicated that even minor dehydration can exacerbate feelings of tension, anxiety, and exhaustion as well as have a detrimental impact on mood.

Brain Health: By promoting appropriate neurotransmitter production and synaptic transmission, adequate hydration promotes brain health and function. As we age, maintaining proper hydration may help avoid cognitive decline and promote general brain health.

Emotional Health and Hydration:

Stress Reduction: By assisting physiological systems that control stress hormones and neurotransmitters, adequate hydration can help lower stress levels and encourage relaxation.

Mood Enhancement: By encouraging sentiments of vigor, optimism, and general well-being, drinking enough water can improve mood and mental health. Conversely, dehydration can make mood swings, irritation, and weariness worse.

Exercise Performance and Hydration:

For optimal performance, both during and after exercise, enough hydration is crucial. Drinking enough water before, during, and after exercise supports energy production, endurance, and muscle function. It also helps prevent dehydration and maintain electrolyte balance.

Temperature regulation: Sweating allows the body to release water and electrolytes when engaging in physical exercise. During exercise, staying hydrated helps avoid overheating, heat exhaustion, and issues connected to dehydration.

Even when you don't feel thirsty, try to consume enough fluids throughout the day to sustain good hydration and promote general wellness. The precise amount of water required varies according on age, body size, degree of activity, climate, and state of health. Aim for 8 to 10 cups (64 to 80 ounces) of water per day as a general guideline, but modify your intake depending on your unique needs and circumstances.

Foods that are high in water content, such as fruits, vegetables, soups, and broths, can also increase the amount of fluid consumed overall. To maintain optimal health and fitness, pay attention to your body's thirst cues and drink water frequently throughout the day. Recall that being well hydrated is a straightforward but crucial habit for fostering general health and energy.

Preventive Medical Care and Examinations

Maintaining general health and wellbeing requires routine screenings and preventive healthcare. People can lessen the burden of disease, improve health outcomes, and improve quality of life by being proactive in preventing sickness, identifying possible health issues early, and managing risk factors. The following are some fundamental ideas of preventive medicine and the significance of screenings:

Frequent Health Check-ups: Make an appointment with your healthcare practitioner on a frequent basis to undergo routine checkups, health assessments, and preventive screenings. Healthcare providers can monitor your health condition, evaluate risk factors, and identify possible health issues early on, when they are most treatable, thanks to these check-ups.

Conduct a thorough health risk assessment to determine personal risk factors for long-term conditions such diabetes, cancer, heart disease, and high blood pressure. Evaluations of lifestyle variables, family history, medical history, and individual health practices are all possible components of health risk assessments.

CHAPTER THREE

Immunizations & Vaccinations: To guard against infectious diseases, stay current on recommended immunizations and vaccinations. Vaccines lower the risk of outbreaks and complications by halting the spread of infectious diseases such the flu, pneumonia, hepatitis, measles, mumps, rubella, and human papillomavirus (HPV).

Preventive screenings and screening tests: Take part in screening tests and preventive measures that are advised in accordance with your age, gender, family history, and personal risk factors. The purpose of screening tests is to identify diseases or problems at an early stage so that treatment and intervention can begin on time. Preventive screenings include, for example:

Cancer Screenings: Early detection of cancer is crucial for the best course of treatment. Regular screenings can help identify common malignancies like breast, cervical, colorectal, prostate, and lung cancer.

Cardiovascular Screenings: Screening tests for cardiovascular disorders, such as electrocardiograms (ECGs), blood pressure checks, and cholesterol checks, can assist determine risk factors for heart disease and stroke as well as examine heart health.

Diabetes Screening: Early detection of diabetes or prediabetes enables lifestyle modifications and preventative actions. Screening tests, such as hemoglobin A1c and fasting blood glucose testing, can aid in this process.

Bone Density Screening: Particularly in postmenopausal women and older persons, bone density scans (DEXA scans) can evaluate bone health and identify osteoporosis or low bone density.

Regular tests for vision and hearing can identify changes in a person's ability to see or hear, which enables early diagnosis and treatment of ocular and ear disorders.

Changes to Your Lifestyle and Health Promotion: Make good choices that will improve your general health and well-being. These include getting regular exercise, eating a balanced diet, managing stress, quitting smoking, using alcohol in moderation, and keeping a healthy weight. By making lifestyle changes and taking preventative steps, health promotion initiatives seek to avoid disease and improve health outcomes.

Patient Education and Empowerment: Become knowledgeable about screening protocols, health promotion tactics, and preventive health suggestions to take an active part in your healthcare. In order to make informed decisions and take proactive measures to prevent sickness and promote wellness, it is important to ask questions, interact with your healthcare practitioner, and advocate for your needs.

People can take charge of their health, lower their risk of disease, and improve their general well-being by emphasizing preventative healthcare and engaging in advised screenings and interventions. Maintaining a healthy lifestyle and living a longer, happier, and more rewarding life are mostly dependent on prevention. It's important to keep in mind that investing in preventive healthcare is an investment in your present and future health, and that starting now will always result in better health outcomes.

Good Practices for Occupational and Environmental Wellness

In order to promote environmental and occupational wellbeing, a supportive and healthful atmosphere must be established in both the workplace and the larger community. People may make a beneficial impact on the environment and foster a pleasant work environment by encouraging habits that put environmental sustainability, workplace safety, and general well-being first. These are some beneficial behaviors for both occupational and environmental wellness:

Sustainability of the Environment:

Reduce, Reuse, Recycle: To cut down on waste and save resources, put the three R's into practice. Minimize your consumption, recycle materials like paper, plastic, glass, and metal, and try to reuse things whenever you can.

Conserve Energy: Make energy-saving appliance and lighting selections, turn off lights and gadgets when not in use, and modify your lifestyle to consume less energy overall.

Use Sustainable Transportation: To cut carbon emissions and advance environmental sustainability, choose eco-friendly modes of transportation wherever you can, such as walking, bicycling, carpooling, or taking public transportation.

Encourage Sustainable Practices: Buy goods and services from businesses that place a high priority on social responsibility and environmental sustainability. Encourage companies to employ renewable energy, reduce waste, and adopt eco-friendly procedures.

Occupational Safety:

Observe Safety standards: To avoid mishaps, injuries, and occupational dangers, abide by workplace safety standards, protocols, and procedures. Learn about safety procedures that are pertinent to your work duties and industry norms.

Wear the Right Gear: To protect yourself from workplace dangers, wear the proper safety gear and personal protection equipment (PPE), such as gloves, goggles, helmets, respirators, and earplugs. Make sure personal protective equipment (PPE) is fitted, maintained, and utilized in accordance with manufacturer guidelines.

Employ ergonomics: To prevent musculoskeletal injuries and to enhance physical comfort and well-being, keep up ergonomic workstations and practices. Modify the arrangement of your desk, furniture, and other items to encourage good posture, lessen strain, and lower your chance of repetitive stress injuries.

Report dangers: As soon as possible, notify your supervisor or other designated safety professionals of any incidents, dangers, or safety concerns. Promote candid dialogue and teamwork to properly handle safety concerns and put preventive measures into place.

Encourage Well-Being

Work-Life Balance: Establish boundaries, give self-care first priority, and schedule time for leisure activities, rest, and relaxation outside of work in order to attain a healthy work-life balance.

Healthy Routines: Include stress-reduction strategies, a balanced diet, frequent exercise, and enough sleep in your everyday schedule. Make mental and physical health a priority to improve productivity, resilience, and general quality of life.

Establish a welcoming and inclusive work atmosphere that encourages cooperation, respect, teamwork, and support among coworkers.

Promote understanding, empathy, and open communication to build a productive and happy work environment.

Advocating for the Environment:

Participate in community projects, volunteer organizations, or environmental advocacy groups that support environmental sustainability, conservation, and eco-friendly behaviors.

Educate and Raise Awareness: To spread knowledge and encourage constructive change, educate others about environmental issues, climate change, and sustainable living techniques. Exchange resources, knowledge, and useful advice on how to reduce carbon footprints and embrace eco-friendly behaviors.

People can improve general well-being in the community and at work, support workplace safety, and contribute to environmental sustainability by adopting these healthy behaviors into their daily lives. Keep in mind that even tiny efforts can have a big impact, and that by working together, we can make the world safer, healthier, and more sustainable for both the present and the future generations.

Developing Coping and Resilience Capabilities

Developing coping mechanisms and resilience is crucial for handling stress, overcoming obstacles in life, and enhancing general wellbeing. The capacity to adjust, recover, and flourish in the face of hardship, disappointments, or major life transitions is known as resilience. People can increase their capacity to handle stressors, boost their mental and emotional resilience, and sharpen their problem-solving abilities by practicing resilience and creating useful coping mechanisms. The following are some essential ideas for developing coping mechanisms and resilience:

Acquire Self-Awareness: To cultivate self-awareness, acknowledge your feelings, ideas, and responses to pressures. Observe how your body and mind react to stress, and note any triggers that can add to overwhelming or distressing feelings.

Gratitude and Hopefulness:

By rephrasing negative ideas and concentrating on solutions rather than problems, you can cultivate optimism and positive thinking. To increase your confidence in your capacity to overcome obstacles, maintain a positive mindset and remind yourself of your prior victories and accomplishments.

Adaptability and Flexibility:

Accept adaptability and flexibility as a way to deal with change and uncertainty. Adopt a growth mentality that sees barriers as chances for learning and development rather than as insurmountable hurdles. Be prepared to modify your expectations, objectives, and goals as necessary to take into account new information.

Look for Social Assistance:

Create a solid support system consisting of friends, family, coworkers, or support groups that can offer consolation, inspiration, and useful help when things go tough. In order to build relationships and get support, reach out to people you can trust and be honest about your needs.

Good Techniques for Solving Problems:

Acquire proficient problem-solving abilities to tackle obstacles and arrive at positive resolutions. Divide difficult issues into smaller, more manageable chunks, come up with ideas for possible fixes, weigh your options, then move to put winning tactics into practice.

Good Coping Strategies:

Develop healthy coping strategies to control your emotions and handle stress. To help you relax and release tension, try deep breathing exercises, mindfulness, progressive muscle relaxation, or meditation.

Take part in fun pursuits and pastimes that make you happy, fulfilled, and proud of yourself. Take time to relax and revitalize by engaging in leisure activities, exploring artistic outlets, or spending time in nature when you're away from stressors.

Set aside time for self-care practices that will support your physical and mental health, such as regular exercise, a healthy diet, enough sleep, and stress reduction methods.

Develop Resilience by Overcoming Adversity:

See adversity as a chance for resilience-building and personal development. Consider previous instances where you overcame difficulties and note the assets, abilities, and strengths that enabled you to manage well. Use these experiences as a source of inspiration and resiliency when things get tough.

If Needed, Seek Professional Assistance:

Do not be afraid to seek professional assistance from a therapist, counselor, or mental health professional if you are having difficulty managing your stress or are suffering severe emotional distress. Effective stress management and resilience building can be greatly aided by the support, direction, and coping mechanisms offered by therapy.

You may build resilience, improve coping mechanisms, and face obstacles in life more confidently and easily by implementing these ideas into your daily life. Resilience is a skill that may be reinforced and developed over time with practice, introspection, and persistence. Developing resilience is a journey, and every step you take in that direction will improve your general well-being and capacity to persevere through hardship.

Engagement in the Social and Community

Engagement in the social and community sphere is essential for creating bonds, establishing relationships, and improving general wellbeing. People can feel a sense of fulfillment, support, and belonging by being involved in the community, volunteering, and socializing. The following are some essential ideas and advantages of social and community involvement:

Improved Social Relationships:

Opportunities to connect with people, form deep connections, and fortify social support networks are presented by social engagement. Social interaction with friends, family, coworkers, and neighbors promotes a feeling of community and togetherness.

Psychological Assistance:

Interacting with people enables the sharing of understanding, empathy, and emotional support in happy, sad, or difficult situations. Talking to trusted people about your experiences, ideas, and feelings can help you feel validated, gain perspective, and find solace.

Decreased Sensations of Alonesomeness and Isolation:

Loneliness and social isolation have been related to poor physical and mental health as well as anxiety and depression. By creating relationships and encouraging a sense of belonging, participating in social activities and community events helps fight feelings of loneliness and isolation.

Enhanced Mental Well-Being:

Participation in social and communal activities has been linked to better mental health outcomes, such as lower stress levels, happier moods, and increased psychological well-being. Engaging in communal endeavors and upholding encouraging connections can enhance self-worth, adaptability, and general contentment with life.

Feeling of Mission and Purpose:

Participating in the community and volunteering offer chances to positively influence others' lives and enhance their well-being. Taking part in worthwhile pursuits that complement one's values and interests helps one feel accomplished, fulfilled, and purposeful.

Improved Well-Being:

Positive physical health outcomes, such as a decreased incidence of chronic illnesses, enhanced immune system performance, and longer life expectancy, have been associated with social support and community involvement. Good social ties and a feeling of community are important for general health and wellbeing.

Personal Development and Skill Development:

Participating in social and community activities presents chances for lifelong learning, personal development, and skill enhancement.

Contributing time to the community, taking part in group activities, and joining groups and organizations can help people learn new things, acquire new skills, and advance personally.

Enhanced ties within the community:

Social and community engagement fosters cooperation, solidarity, and civic engagement, all of which strengthen communities. Community ties are strengthened and a feeling of common identity and purpose is fostered through volunteering for community issues, supporting local initiatives, and taking part in activities.

Encouragement of Equity and Social Justice:

Participation in social and community activities offers forums for promoting inclusion, equity, and social justice. A more just and equitable society can be achieved by individuals through pushing for change, helping marginalized communities, and raising awareness.

Assistance In Times of Need:

Social networks and local resources are vital for helping those in need during catastrophes and times of crisis by offering support, resources, and aid. Resilience and strong communal bonds enable communities to pull together and assist one another through trying times.

People can gain a sense of belonging, support, and social connection by actively engaging in social and community activities. Interacting with others improves our lives and fosters a more dynamic, healthy community, whether via volunteering, joining clubs or groups, going to social events, or funding community projects.

CONCLUSION

To sum up, maintaining one's health requires a holistic approach to wellbeing that takes into account one's physical, mental, emotional, and social needs. People can encourage general health, resilience, and energy by implementing good behaviors and lifestyle routines. The following are some important lessons learned:

Put Your Physical Health First: To promote your physical well-being and fend against sickness, maintain a balanced diet, do regular exercise, drink plenty of water, get enough sleep, and adopt excellent hygiene practices.

Nurture Mental and Emotional Well-Being: To support mental and emotional health, learn stress management strategies, think positively, look for social support, and partake in activities that encourage contentment, joy, and relaxation.

Develop Adaptive Coping Strategies, Encourage Self-Awareness, and Accept Difficulties as Learning and Growth Opportunities to Build Resilience and Coping Skills.

Encourage Social Connections: To encourage a sense of connection, support, and belonging, take part in social and community activities, form dependable connections, and make contributions to the welfare of others.

Embrace Preventive Healthcare: To avoid sickness and encourage early diagnosis of health issues, prioritize preventive healthcare by making frequent check-up appointments, being screened and immunized, and adopting healthy lifestyle practices.

Encourage workplace safety, a good work-life balance, and environmental sustainability to build a community-friendly atmosphere that supports people's individual and collective well-being.

Keep Yourself Informed and Empowered: To make wise decisions and take proactive measures to support your well-being, keep yourself informed about health-related topics, speak up for your needs, and seek expert assistance when necessary.

People can empower themselves to take charge of their health, improve their quality of life, and reap the rewards of leading a meaningful and healthy lifestyle by adopting these ideas into their daily lives. Recall that maintaining your health is a continuous process that calls for resilience, self-care, and commitment; yet, the benefits to your general vitality and well-being make the effort worthwhile.

THE END